HEALTHY HABITS FOR A HEALTHY HEART

Best Natural Preventive Practices For Heart Attack

Robert C. Mansfield

All rights reserved. No part of this publication may be reproduced, distributed, or transmitted in any form or by any means, including photocopying, recording, or other electronic or mechanical methods, without the prior written permission of the publisher, except in the case of brief quotations embodied in critical reviews and certain other noncommercial uses permitted by copyright law. Copyright © Robert C. Mansfield, 2022.

Table of Contents

Chapter One: Heart Attack - What You Need To Know

Chapter Two: Act Fast When You Observe Any Of These Signs

Know What Causes Heart Attack

Chapter Three: Lifestyle Changes For Heart Attack Prevention

Chapter Four: Best Foods You Can Eat To Keep Your Heart Healthy

Chapter One:

Heart Attack - What You Need To Know

A heart attack (medically known as a myocardial infarction) is a severe medical emergency when your heart muscle starts to die because it isn't receiving enough blood flow. This is generally caused by a blockage in the arteries that feed blood to your heart. If blood flow isn't restored soon, a heart attack may cause lasting cardiac damage and death.

A heart attack develops when there is a lack of blood flow to a portion of the heart muscle. It frequently occurs from a blockage in a neighboring artery. A person who is undergoing a heart attack — or myocardial infarction — may experience pain in their chest and other regions of their body, as well as other symptoms.

Spotting the early indications of a heart attack and providing immediate care is vital and can save a person's life.

A cardiac attack is different

Trusted Source from cardiac arrest, in which the heart stops functioning altogether. Both are medical emergencies, and without care, a heart attack may progress to cardiac arrest

Your heart muscle needs a constant supply of oxygen-rich blood. Your coronary arteries offer your heart this crucial blood supply. If you have coronary artery disease, those arteries grow narrow, and blood can't flow as well as it should. When your blood supply is blocked, you suffer a heart attack.

Fat, calcium, proteins, and inflammatory cells pile up in your arteries to create plaques. These plaque deposits are firm on the exterior and soft and mushy on the inside.

When the plaque gets firm, the outer shell fractures. This is termed a rupture. Platelets (disc-shaped items in your blood that help it clot) arrive at the location, and blood clots form around the plaque. If a blood clot stops your artery, your heart muscle becomes starving for oxygen. The muscle cells quickly die, causing lasting injury.

Rarely, a spasm in your coronary artery might potentially induce a heart attack. During this coronary spasm, your arteries constrict or spasm on and off, cutting off the blood flow to your heart muscle (ischemia) (ischemia). It can happen when you're at rest and even if you don't have substantial coronary artery disease.

Each coronary artery supplies blood to a distinct area of your heart muscle. How much the muscle is harmed relies on the size of the region that the blocked artery serves and the length of time between the attack and therapy.

Your heart muscle begins to repair immediately after a heart attack. This takes roughly 8 weeks. Just like a flesh wound, a scar grows in the affected region. But the new scar tissue doesn't move the way it should. So your heart can't pump as much after a heart attack. How much that ability to pump is affected depends on the size and location of the scar.

What Do I Do if I Have A Heart Attack?

After a heart attack, you need quick treatment to open the blocked artery and lessen the damage. At the first signs of a heart attack, call 911. The best time to treat a heart attack is within 1 or 2 hours after symptoms begin. Waiting longer means more damage to your heart and a lower chance of survival.

If you've phoned emergency services and are waiting for them to come, eat an aspirin (325 mg). Aspirin is a powerful inhibitor of blood clots and may cut the risk of mortality from a heart attack by 25%.

What Do I Do if Someone Else Has A Heart Attack?

Call 911 and start CPR (cardiopulmonary resuscitation) if someone goes into cardiac arrest, which is when the heartbeat has stopped and the individual isn't responsive. CPR doesn't restart the heart; rather it keeps the victim alive until medical aid comes.

An easy-to-use gadget called an AED (automated external defibrillator) is accessible in many public areas and may be used by nearly anybody to treat cardiac arrest. This gadget operates by shocking the heart back into a regular rhythm.

Here's how to use an AED:

1. Check responsiveness

For an adult or older kid, yell and shake the individual to establish if they're unconscious. Do not use AED on a conscious individual.
For a newborn or young kid, squeeze their skin. Never shake a tiny kid.
Check breathing and pulse. If missing or unequal, prepare to use the AED as soon as feasible.

2. Prepare to utilize AED

Make sure the individual is in a dry environment and away from puddles or water.
Check for body piercings or outline of an implanted medical device, such as a pacemaker or implantable defibrillator.
AED pads must be positioned at least 1 inch away from piercings or implanted devices.

3. Use AED

For newborns, babies, and children up to age 8, utilize a pediatric AED, if feasible. If not, use an adult AED.

- Turn on the AED.
- Wipe the chest dry.
- Attach pads.
- Plug-in connection, if required.
- Make sure no one is touching the individual.
- Push the "Analyze" button.
- If a shock is indicated, check again to make sure no one is touching the victim.
- Push the "Shock" button.
- Start or resume continuing compressions.
- Follow AED instructions.

4. Continue CPR

After 2 minutes of CPR, check the person's heart rhythm. If it's still missing or inconsistent, give them another shock.

If a shock isn't required, continue CPR until emergency aid comes or the victim starts to move. Stay with the individual until aid comes.

Why Should I Take Part In Cardiac Rehabilitation?

If you've had a heart attack or have been diagnosed with heart disease, your doctor may suggest cardiac rehabilitation. You'll work with a team of professionals to increase your health and prevent future difficulties.

Your team may include physicians and nurses, as well as experts in exercise, nutrition, physical therapy, occupational therapy, and mental health. They'll build up a program to match your requirements. They may also assist you to make adjustments in your everyday life. If you stay with it, it may make a tremendous impact on your recuperation and general well

Chapter Two:

Act Fast When You Observe Any Of These Signs

Symptoms of a heart attack include:

Discomfort, pressure, weight, tightness, squeezing, or pain in your chest or arm or below your breastbone

Discomfort that goes into your back, jaw, neck, or arm, fullness, indigestion, or a choking sensation (it may feel like heartburn), sweating, upset stomach, vomiting, or dizziness, severe weakness, anxiety, weariness, or shortness of breath, Fast or irregular heartbeat.

Symptoms might be variable from person to person or from one heart attack to another. Women are more likely to experience these heart attack symptoms:

- Unusual tiredness
- Shortness of breath
- Nausea or vomiting
- Dizziness or lightheadedness
- Discomfort in your stomach. It may feel like indigestion.
- Discomfort in the neck, shoulder, or upper back

With some heart attacks, you won't notice any symptom (a "silent" myocardial infarction). This is more likely in those who have diabetes.

Angina

Angina isn't a condition or sickness. It's a symptom, and occasionally it might suggest a heart attack. The symptoms may occur with

typical activity or effort but then go away with rest or when you take nitroglycerin.
You may feel:

- Pressure, soreness, squeezing, or a sensation of fullness in the middle of the chest
- Pain or discomfort in the shoulder, arm, back, neck, or jaw

Call 911 if it grows worse, lasts longer than 5 minutes, or doesn't improve after you've taken nitroglycerin. Doctors term it "unstable" angina," and it's an emergency that might be tied to a heart attack that is about to happen.

If you instead have "stable" angina, which is the most frequent variety, your symptoms generally arise with known triggers (such as a strong emotion, physical activity, severe hot and cold conditions, or even a large meal) (such as a strong emotion, physical activity, extreme hot and cold temperatures, or even a heavy meal). The symptoms go away if you relax or take the nitroglycerin that your doctor has given you. If not, call 911.

The symptoms might vary in their sequence and length – they may last several days or arrive and go unexpectedly.

The following may also develop:

Hypoxemia: This includes low amounts of oxygen in the blood.

Pulmonary edema: This involves fluid accumulating in and around the lungs.

Cardiogenic shock: This includes blood pressure lowering abruptly because the heart cannot deliver enough blood for the rest of the body to perform effectively.

Know What Causes Heart Attack

Coronary artery disease causes most heart attacks. In coronary artery disease, one or more of the heart (coronary) arteries are clogged. This is mainly caused by cholesterol-containing deposits called plaques. Plaques may restrict the arteries, limiting blood flow to the heart.

If a plaque bursts open, it might create a blood clot in the heart.

A heart attack may be caused by a total or partial blockage of a heart (coronary) artery. One approach to identify heart attacks is whether an electrocardiogram (ECG or EKG) exhibits any particular abnormalities (ST elevation) that necessitate emergent invasive treatment. Your health care physician may use ECG readings to define various kinds of heart attacks.

An immediate full blockage of a medium or large cardiac artery typically signifies you've suffered an ST elevation myocardial infarction (STEMI).

A partial blockage frequently suggests you've suffered a non-ST elevation myocardial infarction (NSTEMI). However, some persons with NSTEMI have a complete obstruction.
Not all heart attacks are caused by clogged arteries. Other factors include:

Coronary artery spasm. This is a strong squeezing of a blood artery that's not obstructed. The artery typically contains cholesterol plaques or there is early hardening of the vessel owing to smoking or other risk factors. Other terms for coronary artery spasms include Prinzmetal's angina, vasospastic angina, or variant angina.
Certain infections. COVID-19 and other viral infections may cause damage to the heart muscle.

Spontaneous coronary artery dissection (SCAD) (SCAD). This life-threatening illness is caused by a tear within a cardiac artery

Heart attacks are triggered by the blood flow to the heart being unexpectedly disrupted. Without this supply, cardiac muscles may be injured and begin to die. Without therapy, the cardiac muscles will incur irreparable damage.

If a major section of the heart is injured in this manner, the heart stops beating (known as a cardiac arrest), ending in death.

Coronary Heart Disease

Coronary heart disease (CHD) is the major cause of heart attacks. CHD is a disorder in which the coronary arteries (the primary blood vessels that supply the heart with blood) become blocked with deposits of cholesterol. These deposits are termed plaques.

Before a heart attack, one of the plaques ruptures (bursts), causing a blood clot to develop at the site of the rupture. The clot may obstruct the supply of blood to the heart, prompting a heart attack.

Your chance of acquiring CHD is enhanced by: smoking, high-fat, diabetes, high cholesterol, high blood pressure (hypertension), being overweight or obese

Less Common Causes

Some less frequent reasons are discussed below.

Drug Abuse

Using stimulants such as cocaine, amphetamines (speed) and methamphetamines (crystal meth) may cause coronary arteries to constrict, reducing blood circulation and precipitating a heart attack.

Heart attack from the usage of cocaine is one of the most prevalent reasons for sudden mortality in young individuals.

Lack Of Oxygen In The Blood (Hypoxia)

If levels of oxygen in the blood decline owing to carbon monoxide poisoning or a lack of normal lung function, the heart will get un-oxygenated blood.

This will result in the heart muscles being destroyed, prompting a heart attack.

Chapter Three:

Lifestyle Changes For Heart Attack Prevention

Sounds easy, doesn't it? Heart disease is the No. 1 cause of death in the United States. Stroke is the No. 5 cause of mortality in the United States.

One of the largest factors to these figures is a lack of dedication to a heart-healthy lifestyle. Your lifestyle is not just your greatest protection against heart disease and stroke, it's also your duty. A heart-healthy lifestyle comprises the concepts mentioned below. By following these easy actions you may minimize all of the modifiable risk factors for heart disease, heart attack, and stroke.

Lifestyle Changes

Know Your Risk

If you're between 40 and 75 years old and have never had a heart attack or stroke, utilize the Check. Change. Control. calculator to assess your risk of having a cardiovascular incident in the following 10 years. Certain factors may raise your risks, such as smoking, renal illness, or a family history of early heart disease. Knowing your risk factors may help you and your health care team decide on the best treatment option for you. Many risk factors may be addressed with lifestyle adjustments.

Stop Smoking

If you smoke, quit. If someone in your home smokes, urge them to stop. We realize it's challenging. But it's difficult to recover after a heart attack or stroke or to live with chronic heart disease. Commit to quitting.

Choose Proper Nutrition

A balanced diet is one of the finest tools you have to battle the cardiovascular disease. The food you consume (and the quantity) may impact other controllable risk factors: cholesterol, blood pressure, diabetes, and overweight. Choose nutrient-rich foods — which include vitamins, minerals, fiber, and other nutrients but are lower in calories — over nutrient-poor meals. Choose a diet that promotes consumption of vegetables, fruits, and whole grains; includes low-fat dairy products, chicken, fish, legumes, nontropical vegetable oils, and nuts; and restricts the intake of sweets, and sugar-sweetened drinks, and red meats. And to maintain a healthy weight, coordinate your food with your physical activity level so you're using up as many calories as you take in.

Learn How To Eat Healthily.

High blood cholesterol

Fat stuck in your arteries is a nightmare waiting to happen. Sooner or later it might produce a heart attack or stroke. You've got to limit your diet of saturated fat, trans fat, and cholesterol and begin active. If food and physical exercise alone don't bring those levels down, then medication may be the solution. Take it precisely how the doctor prescribes. Here's the rundown on where those numbers need to be:

Total Cholesterol

Your total cholesterol score is computed using the following equation: HDL + LDL + 20 percent of your triglyceride level.

Low-density-lipoprotein (LDL) cholesterol = "bad" cholesterol

A low LDL cholesterol level is considered favorable for your heart health. However, your LDL score should no longer be the major consideration in directing therapy to avoid heart attack and stroke, according to the current recommendations from the American Heart Association. For individuals using statins, the recommendations suggest they no longer need to bring LDL cholesterol levels down to a specified target amount. Lifestyle variables such as a diet heavy in saturated and fats may boost LDL cholesterol.

High-density-lipoprotein (HDL) cholesterol = "good" cholesterol

With HDL (good) cholesterol, greater levels are normally preferable. Low HDL cholesterol puts you at increased risk for heart disease. People with high blood triglycerides frequently also have reduced HDL cholesterol. Genetic factors, type 2 diabetes, smoking, being overweight, and being sedentary may all result in reduced HDL cholesterol

Triglycerides

Triglyceride is the most frequent form of fat in the body. Normal triglyceride levels vary by age and sex. A high triglyceride level paired with low HDL cholesterol or high LDL cholesterol is connected with atherosclerosis, the development of fatty deposits in artery walls that raises the risk for heart attack and stroke.

Lower high blood pressure

It's a key risk factor for stroke a leading cause of disability in the United States. Stroke rehabilitation is challenging at best and you might be crippled for life. Shake that salt habit, take your meds as suggested by your doctor and begin exercising. Those numbers need to go down and remain low. An optimum blood pressure value is less than 120/80 mmHg.

Be Physically Active Every Day

Be physically active every day. Research has indicated that at least 150 minutes per week of moderate-intensity physical exercise may help decrease blood pressure, lower cholesterol, and maintain your weight at a healthy level. And anything IS better than nothing. If you're inactive currently, start gradually. Even a few minutes at a time may bring some health advantages. Studies reveal that those who have reached even a modest degree of fitness are substantially less likely to die early than those with a poor fitness level.

Aim Towards A Healthy Weight

Obesity is increasingly widespread in America, not just for adults but also for youngsters. Fad diets and supplements are not the solutions. A good diet, regulating calorie consumption, and physical exercise are the only way to maintain a healthy weight. Obesity puts you at risk for high cholesterol, high blood pressure, and insulin resistance, a forerunner of type 2 diabetes – the same characteristics that heighten your risk of cardiovascular disease. Your Body Mass Index (BMI) may assist inform you whether your weight is healthy.

Manage Diabetes

At least 68% of those 65 years of age with DM die of some kind of HD; 16% die of stroke. Other risk factors, such as high blood pressure, high cholesterol, smoking, obesity, and lack of physical exercise may dramatically increase a person with diabetes' probability of getting cardiovascular disease.

Reduce Stress

A few studies have observed a link between coronary heart disease risk and stress in a person's life that may impact the risk factors for heart disease and stroke. For example, persons under stress may overeat, start smoking or smoke more than they normally would. Research has even demonstrated that stress response in young individuals predicts middle-age blood pressure risk.

Limit Alcohol

Drinking too much alcohol may elevate blood pressure, promote cardiomyopathy, stroke, cancer, and other disorders It may lead to excessive triglycerides and induce irregular heartbeats. Excessive alcohol intake causes obesity, alcoholism, suicide, and accidents.

However, there is a cardioprotective benefit of moderate alcohol use. If you drink, restrict your alcohol intake to no more than two drinks per day for males and no more than one drink per day for women. The National Institute on Alcohol Abuse and Alcoholism defines a drink as 1-1/2 fluid ounces (fl oz) of 80-proof spirits (such as bourbon, Scotch, vodka, gin, etc.), 5 fl oz of wine, or 12 fl oz of regular beer. It's not suggested that nondrinkers start using alcohol or that drinkers increase the quantity they drink.

Saving Lives One Step At A Time

How can being physically active today affect your heart health down the road? With the assistance of modern technologies like the Apple Watch and iPhones, researchers are examining the relationship and generating advancements that can help us all enjoy longer, healthier lives.

Recovery from a cardiac issue becomes so much more doable when you have the correct type of emotional support. We're an online community of patients, survivors, and caregivers who know what you're going through and can help you find your footing on the journey to better health.

Take Your Meds.

If you have a health issue, your doctor may prescribe statins or other drugs to help reduce cholesterol, blood sugar, and blood pressure. Take all drugs as prescribed. But don't use aspirin as a prophylactic step unless your doctor instructs you to. If you've never had a heart attack or stroke, daily aspirin may not assist you at all and might create complications like the danger of bleeding. If you've had a heart attack or stroke, your doctor may want you to take a low dosage of aspirin to lower your chance of having another.

Be A Team Player.

Your health care team can help you minimize your risk of heart disease or stroke to live a longer, healthier life. Work together on your preventative strategy. Ask questions, and be candid about any problems you may experience in attempting to make healthy changes. Stress, sleep, mental health, familial difficulties, cigarette use, food availability, social support, and other concerns all influence your health and well-being.

Live Properly Now For A Healthier Future.

The bottom line? Healthy living is the greatest approach to preventing or avoiding many heart and brain problems. This involves being active and fit, eating healthy, avoiding cigarettes, and treating diseases that may put you at increased risk. Take control of your health. Join Healthy for Good for advice, resources, and motivation to make changes and develop healthy habits you can continue throughout your life.

Chapter Four:

Best Foods You Can Eat To Keep Your Heart Healthy

How can you enhance your heart health with food?

There are several things you can do to help keep your heart healthy and disease-free. You may arrange an annual checkup, exercise every day, stop smoking, or take efforts to lessen the amount of stress in your life.

All of these items may have a favorable influence on heart health. But, one of the easiest lifestyle modifications that can assist your heart is minding what you eat. Nearly 6 million trusted Source persons are presently living with heart failure, and over half of them will die within 5 years of being diagnosed.

The Centers for Disease Control and Prevention (CDC) advise that consuming meals heavy in fat, cholesterol, or salt may be highly dangerous for the heart. So, when taking action to limit the risk of heart disease, nutrition is a smart place to start.

In this book, we analyze some of the finest foods for ensuring that you retain a strong and healthy heart.

Foods That Can Save Your Heart

Fresh Herbs

When you add them to dishes instead of salt and fat, you're making a heart-healthy option. They provide taste without the nasty things. Spices and other foods are excellent ways to eat heart-smart.

Black Beans

Mild, delicate black beans are rich in heart-healthy minerals. Folate, antioxidants, and magnesium may help decrease blood pressure. Their fiber helps regulate both cholesterol and blood sugar levels. Add beans to enrich soups and salads.

Prep Tip: Rinse canned beans to eliminate excess salt.

Red Wine with Resveratrol

If you consume alcohol, a little red wine may be a heart-healthy decision. Resveratrol and catechins, two antioxidants in red wine, may protect arterial walls. Alcohol may also enhance HDL, the healthy cholesterol.

Tip: Too much alcohol harms the heart. Don't have more than one drink a day for ladies or two drinks for males. It's wise to chat to your doctor first. Alcohol may create issues for persons using aspirin and other medicines.

Salmon: Super Food

A top meal for heart health, it's high in omega-3s. Omega-3s are beneficial fats that may minimize the risk of cardiac rhythm problems and lower blood pressure. They may also decrease triglycerides and prevent inflammation. The American Heart Association advises two meals of salmon or other fatty fish a week.

Cooking Tip: Bake fish in foil with herbs and vegetables. Toss additional cooked salmon in fish tacos and salads.

Tuna for Omega-3s

Often cheaper than salmon, tuna also provides omega-3s. Albacore (white tuna) contains higher omega-3s than other tuna kinds. Try grilling tuna steak with dill and lemon. Reel in these additional sources of omega-3s, too: mackerel, herring, lake trout, sardines, and anchovies.

Health Tip: Choose tuna packaged in water, not oil, to keep it heart-healthy.

Olive Oil

This oil is a healthy fat derived from crushed olives. It's high in heart-healthy antioxidants. They may protect your blood vessels. When olive oil substitutes saturated fat (like butter), it may help decrease cholesterol levels. Try it on salads and cooked vegetables, or toast.

Taste tip: For the finest taste, go for cold-pressed and utilize it within 6 months.

Walnuts

A mere handful of walnuts a day may decrease your cholesterol. It may also protect against inflammation in your heart's arteries. Walnuts are filled with omega-3s, healthy fats called monounsaturated fats, plant sterols, and fiber. The advantages arise when walnuts substitute harmful fats, such as those in chips and cookies.

Tip: Try walnut oil in salad dressings.

Almonds

Slivered almonds work nicely with vegetables, fish, poultry, and sweets. They contain plant sterols, fiber, and heart-healthy fats. Almonds may help lower "bad" LDL cholesterol. Grab a tiny handful a day.

Taste Tip: Toast them to increase their creamy, mild taste.

Edamame

You may have seen them as an appetizer at an Asian restaurant. Edamame is the Japanese term for soybeans. Soy protein may help decrease cholesterol levels. A cup of edamame also provides 8 grams of heart-healthy fiber. To acquire that much fiber from whole wheat bread, you'd need to consume around four pieces.

Tip: Take frozen edamame, boil it, and then serve warm in the pod. Popping out the yummy beans from the tough pod makes a satisfying snack.

Tofu

Eat tofu and you'll receive a superb source of vegetarian soy protein with heart-healthy minerals, fiber, and polyunsaturated fats. It may take on the flavor of the spices or sauces you use to prepare it.

Tips: Chop firm tofu, marinade, then grill or stir-fry, going low on the oil. Add tofu to soups for protein with minimum additional oil.

Sweet Potatoes

Swap white potatoes with sweet potatoes. With a lower glycemic index than white potatoes, these spuds won't trigger a fast surge in blood sugar. They also include fiber, vitamin A, and lycopene.

Taste Tip: Boost their natural sweetness with a sprinkling of cinnamon and lime juice instead of sugary toppings.

Oranges

Sweet and juicy, oranges offer the cholesterol-fighting fiber pectin. They also include potassium, which helps manage blood pressure. In one research, 2 glasses of OJ a day enhanced blood vessel health. It also decreased blood pressure in males.

Nutrition Tip: A medium orange offers around 62 calories and 3 grams of fiber.

Swiss Chard

This dark green, leafy vegetable is rich in potassium and magnesium. These minerals assist manage blood pressure. Swiss chard also has heart-healthy fiber, vitamin A, and the antioxidants lutein and zeaxanthin. Try serving it with grilled meats or as a bed for fish.

Prep Tip: Sauté it with olive oil and garlic until wilted. Season with herbs and pepper.

Barley

Try this nutty whole grain instead of rice. You may also cook barley into soups and stews. The fiber in barley may help decrease cholesterol levels. It may reduce blood sugar levels, too.

Tip: Get to know your barley. Hulled or "whole grain" barley is the most nutritious. Barley grits are roasted and ground. They make a delicious cereal or as a side dish. Pearl barley is fast, but a lot of the heart-healthy fiber has been eliminated.

Oatmeal

A warm cup of oatmeal fills you full for hours, resists snack attacks, and helps maintain blood sugar levels steady over time — making it valuable for those with diabetes, too. Oats' fiber may aid your heart by decreasing harmful cholesterol (LDL) (LDL). Best results come from utilizing steel cut or slow-cooked oats.

Baking Tip: Making pancakes, muffins, or other baked goods? Swap out one-third of the flour and put in oats instead.

Flaxseed

This lustrous, honey-colored seed offers three things that are excellent for your heart: fiber, phytonutrients called lignans, and omega-3 fatty acids.

Tip: Grind flaxseed for the finest nutrients. Add it to cereal, baked goods, yogurt, or mustard on a sandwich.

Low-Fat Yogurt

When you think of dairy foods, you probably think, "Good for my bones!" These meals may help lower high blood pressure, too. Yogurt is rich in calcium and potassium. To fully enhance the calcium and decrease the fat, pick low-fat kinds.

Foods Fortified With Sterols

Some kinds of margarine, soy milk, almond milk, and orange juices have cholesterol-fighting sterols and stanols added. These plant ingredients inhibit your intestines from absorbing cholesterol. They can cut LDL levels by 10% without affecting good cholesterol.

Cherries

Sweet cherries, sour cherries, dry cherries, and cherry juice — they're all excellent. All are filled with antioxidants called anthocyanins. They're supposed to help protect blood arteries.

Get More: Sprinkle dried cherries into cereal, muffin batter, green salads, and wild rice.

Blueberries

Blueberries are fantastic when it comes to nutrients. They've got anthocyanins, those blood vessel-helping antioxidants. Those antioxidants give the berries their rich blue hue. Blueberries also offer fiber and more than a handful of other important nutrients. Add fresh or dried blueberries to cereal, pancakes, or yogurt.

Dessert Idea: Puree a batch for a sweet sauce you can use as a dip or pour on other sweet desserts.

Dark Leafy Greens

Your folks were onto something when they encouraged you to eat your greens. They're packed with vitamins and minerals. They're also high in nitrates, a substance that helps to open blood vessels so oxygen-rich blood can reach your heart. You'll find them in vegetables like:

Serving tip: Bring out the taste by adding greens to a stir-fry, sauté them with olive oil, or roast them with garlic.

Garlic

When you spice up your meals, you could also safeguard your heart. People have used garlic as medicine for millennia, and research on supplements suggests it may have advantages for your blood pressure and cholesterol levels. Talk to your doctor before you try any pills, since it may raise your risk of bleeding and interfere with the meds you take.

Green Tea

Drink plenty if you want to minimize your risk of heart disease and stroke. Research shows that compounds in it called catechins may decrease your cholesterol. If you're not a lover of this drink, it also comes in pill form, but consult your doctor first..

Pectin

Fruits such as apples and strawberries offer this kind of soluble fiber, which helps decrease your LDL cholesterol. Although you may also take it as a supplement, health experts suggest eating is ideal.

Soy

Tweak your diet and incorporate items produced from this plant in the pea family. Some possibilities include edamame, soy milk, and tofu. They'll assist your heart if you consume them instead of meat that's heavy in fat.

Pomegranate

This fruit is a potent antioxidant that may help keep your arteries clean and protect your heart. Some people appreciate its tangy taste, but if it's not for you and you want to take a supplement, check with your doctor. Pills don't combine well with certain medications.

Asparagus

Asparagus is a natural source of folate, which helps to prevent an amino acid called homocysteine from building up in the body. High homocysteine levels have been connected with trusted Sources an increased risk of heart-related diseases, such as coronary artery disease and stroke.

Beans, peas, chickpeas, and lentils

Beans, peas, chickpeas, and lentils — sometimes known as pulses or legumes — may all considerably lower levels of low-density lipoprotein (LDL) or "bad cholesterol." They are also rich in fiber, protein, and antioxidant polyphenols, all of which have good benefits for the heart and overall health.

Berries

Berries are also abundant in antioxidant polyphenols, which aid to decrease heart disease Trusted Source risk. Berries are a fantastic source of fiber, folate, iron, calcium, vitamin A, and vitamin C, and they are low in fat.

Broccoli.

Some research shows that routinely eating steamed broccoli helps decrease cholesterol levels and preventTrusted Source heart disease.

Chia seeds and flaxseeds

These seeds are a high plant-based source of omega-3 fatty acids, such as alpha-linolenic acid rusted Source. Omega-3s have several positive benefits, such as helping to reduce levels of triglycerides, LDL, and total cholesterol. They also lower blood pressure and limit the formation of fatty plaques in the arteries.

Dark chocolate

Dark chocolate is a rare example of a meal that tastes fantastic and is beneficial for you (in moderation) (in moderation).

Dark chocolate: delicious and heart-healthy. Scientists now think that dark chocolate provides preventive advantages against atherosclerosis, which is when plaque builds up within the arteries, raising the risk of heart attack and stroke.

Dark chocolate appears to inhibit two of the processes involved in atherosclerosis: stiffness of the arteries and white blood cell adhesion, which is when white blood cells cling to the walls of blood vessels.

What is more, studies have revealed that increasing dark chocolate's flavanol concentration — which is the component that makes it sweet and moreish — does not lessen these protective advantages.

Coffee

Also in the "almost too wonderful to be true" category is coffee. One recent research indicated that frequently consuming coffee was connected with a lower risk trusted Source of having heart failure and stroke.

However, it is vital to keep in mind that this research — which employed machine learning to examine data from the Framingham Heart Study — can only notice a relationship between characteristics, and cannot prove cause and effect.

Liver

Of all the organ meats, the liver is the most nutrient-dense. In particular, the liver is bulging with folic acid, iron, chromium, copper, and zinc, which increase the blood's hemoglobin level and help to keep our heart healthy.

Spinach

You can help to maintain a healthy heart rhythm by regularly consuming good sources of magnesium. Spinach is one of the best sources of dietary magnesium, and consumption of Popeye's favorite food is associated with a raft of health benefits.

Tomatoes

Tomatoes have lots of nutrients that might help keep our hearts healthy. The small red fruits are chock-full of fiber, potassium, vitamin C, folate, and choline, which are all excellent for the heart.

As well as helping to keep heart disease at bay, potassium improves muscles and bones and helps prevent kidney stones from developing.

Scientists have claimed that increasing potassium Trusted Source consumption while lowering salt intake is the most essential dietary modification when aiming to minimize the risk of heart disease.

Vegetables

The AHA recommended that we consume eight or more trusted Source portions of fruit and vegetables each day. Vegetables are low in fat and calories but rich in fiber, minerals, and vitamins. A healthful amount of veggies in the diet can help to moderate weight and blood pressure.

www.ingramcontent.com/pod-product-compliance
Lightning Source LLC
Chambersburg PA
CBHW050312220526
45465CB00005B/1959